Acknowledgement

I would like to thank my family, friends and mentors for your love and support on my second book in the series. I'd also like to give a special thank you to my beautiful grandchildren, Amiya Ferrell, Calvin Ferrell Jr, Trey Ferrell and Khai Ferrell. Your beautiful smiles inspire NaNa everyday.

Dedication

I would like to dedicate this second book to my three sons. Mark, I love your confidence, leadership skills and the way you always love and respect me. You have never let me down. Calvin, I love your heart, your love for me and your giving spirit. You will give the shirt off of your back to a total stranger if they needed it. Lydell, I love your intellect, strength, perseverance and how you show your love for me everyday. You have never been a follower. Quote: God uses ordinary people to do the most extraordinary things.

Amiya woke up ready to start her day,

but not before brushing her teeth.

She opened her magical box and out

jumped Brushy and Squeezy.

"Hello," she greeted them as her face lit up.

"Are you ready to start brushing?"

Brushy asked Amiya.

"Ready and waiting,"

Amiya responded.

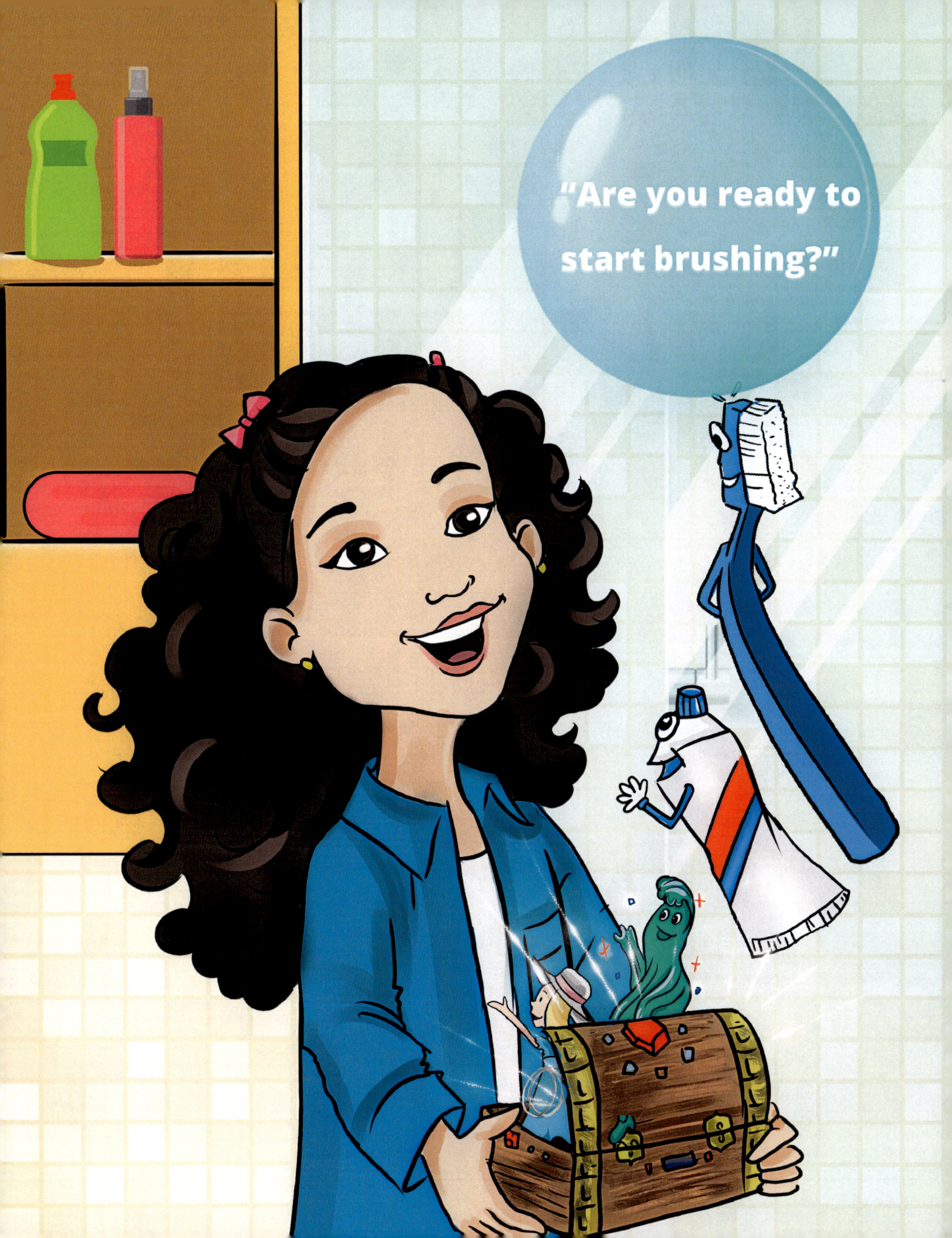

It's time to floss first," said Flossy. Flossy jumped up and started to spin her lasso of dental floss. Amiya grasped hold and started to floss. "From front to back, and back to front, this is the way we get rid of the gunk!" Flossy sang

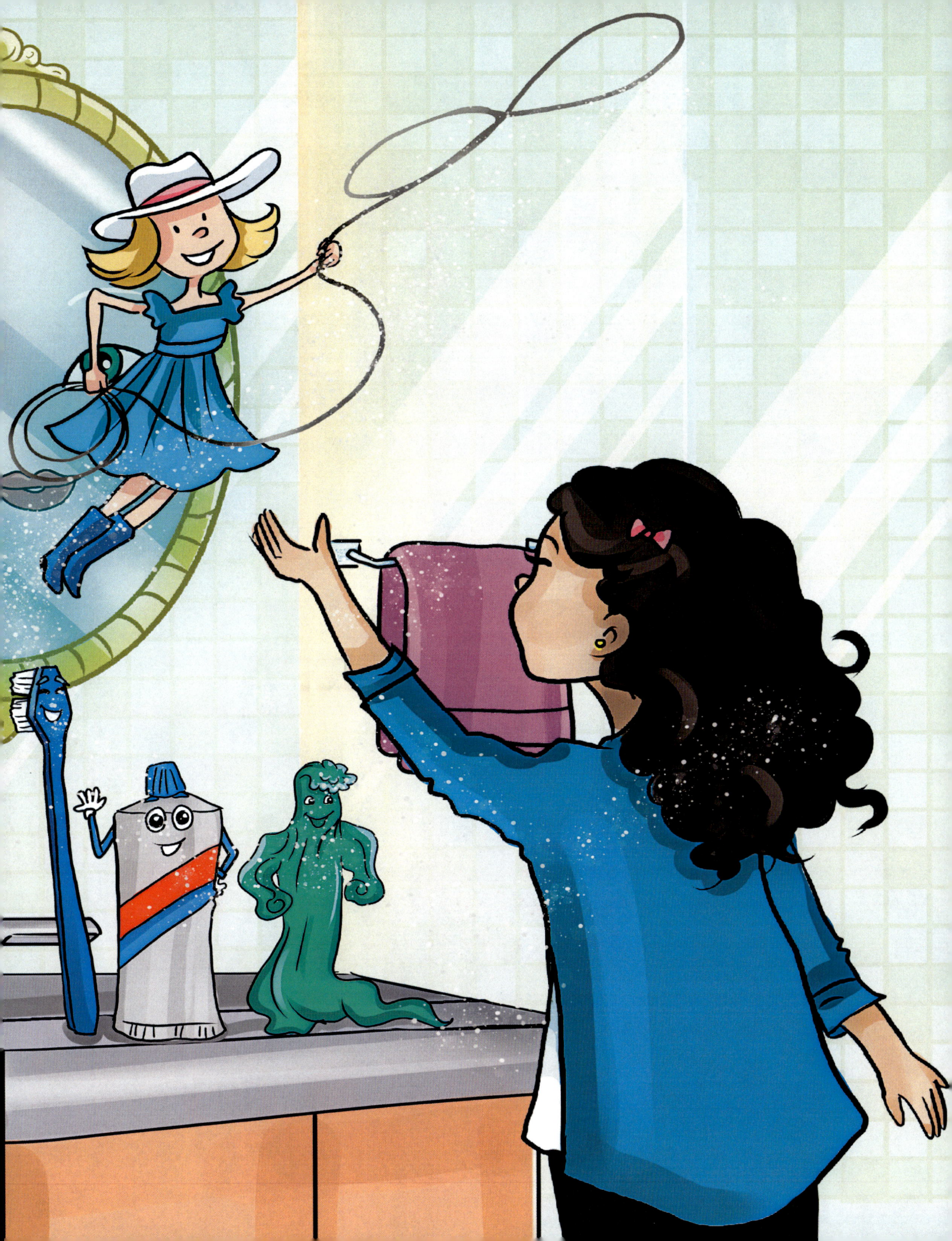

"Now it's time to brush," said Brushy. Because of Amiya's two-minute timer on Brushy, Amiya knew exactly when to stop brushing, and she did just that as soon as it started to beep

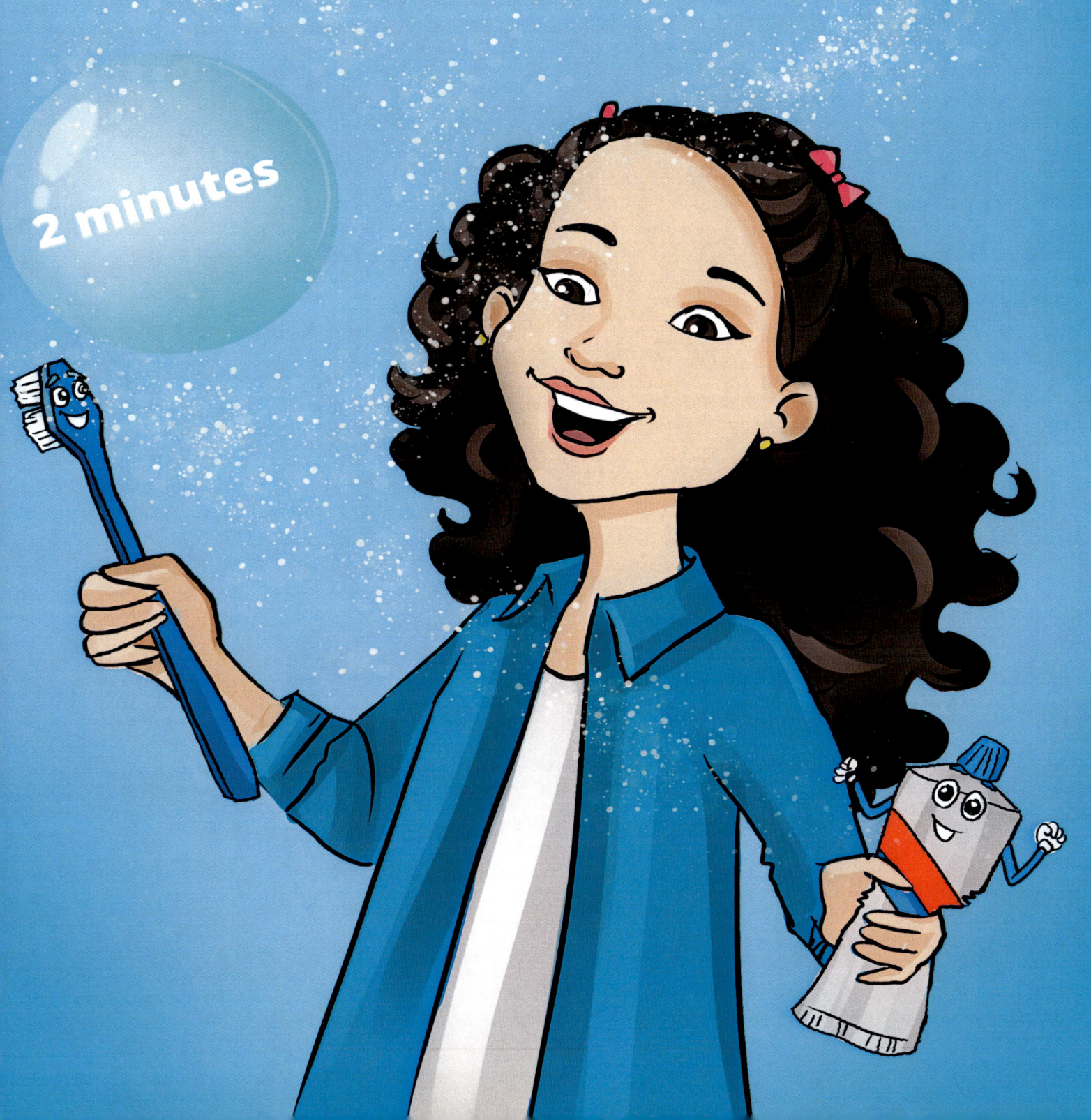

"Now it's time to rinse with fluoride," Amiya said. "I like to do this every day to help keep my teeth healthy and strong." Then, Flouri started to glow and sparkle, and he poured just enough fluoride into his cap for Amiya to use. Flouri sang while Amiya swished. "From front to back, and back to front, swishing is such fun, fun, fun!"

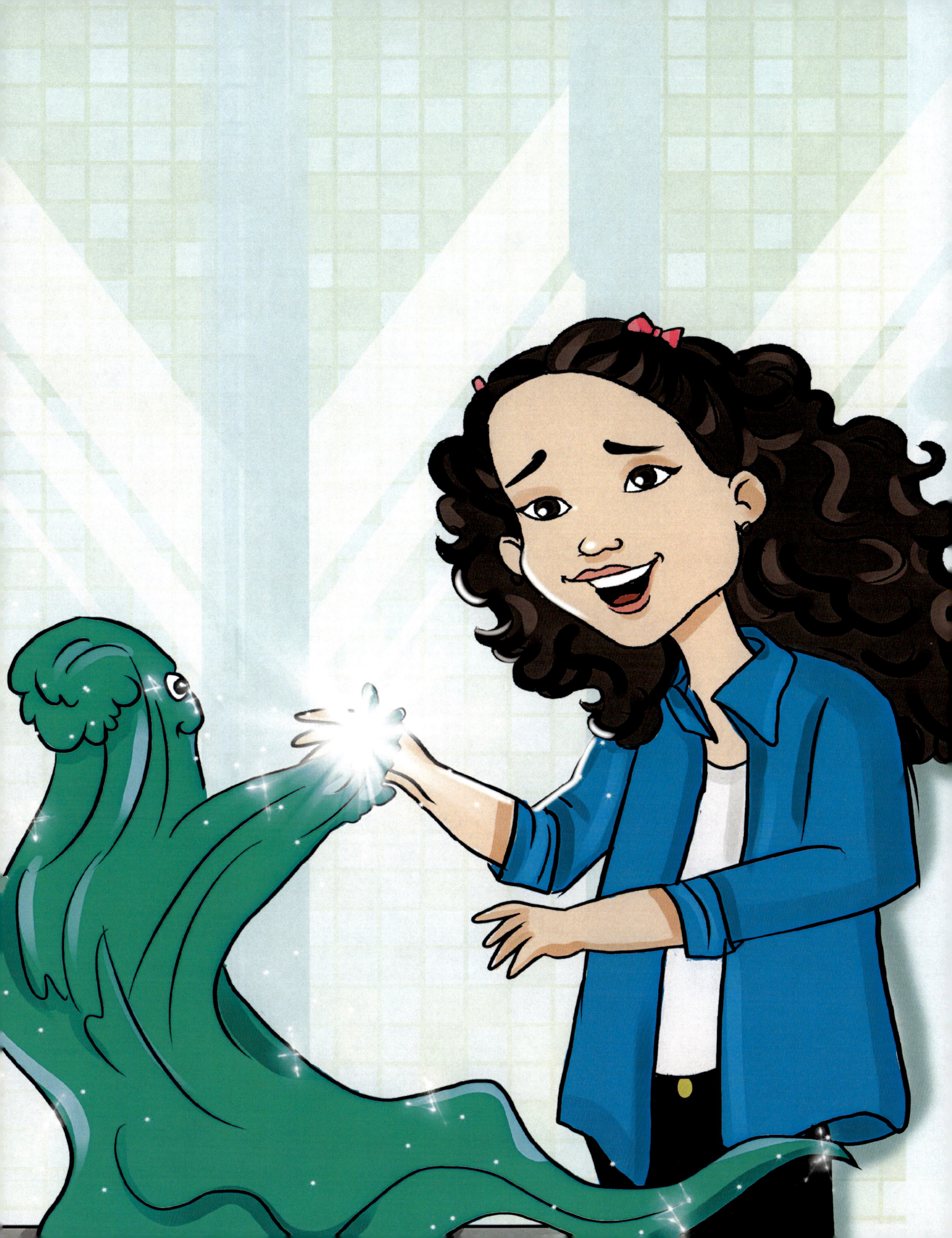

Just then Maggy the magical mirror started to shimmer and shine.

"Hello" said Maggy the magical mirror.

"Hello Maggy," they all said together.

"Oh no!" Maggy suddenly exclaimed. She was wearing a strange look on her face "What's the matter?" Amiya asked

There is a boy named Anthony who did not brush his teeth today," Maggy replied. "Why didn't he brush his teeth today?" Amiya asked.

"Anthony thinks that just because he brushed his teeth last night, that it's okay to go without brushing them today," Maggy explained.

"That is a bad idea," Brushy added. "What Anthony doesn't know is that if he doesn't brush his teeth twice per day every day, his teeth will get covered with plaque and bacteria, which makes it easier for him to get cavities."

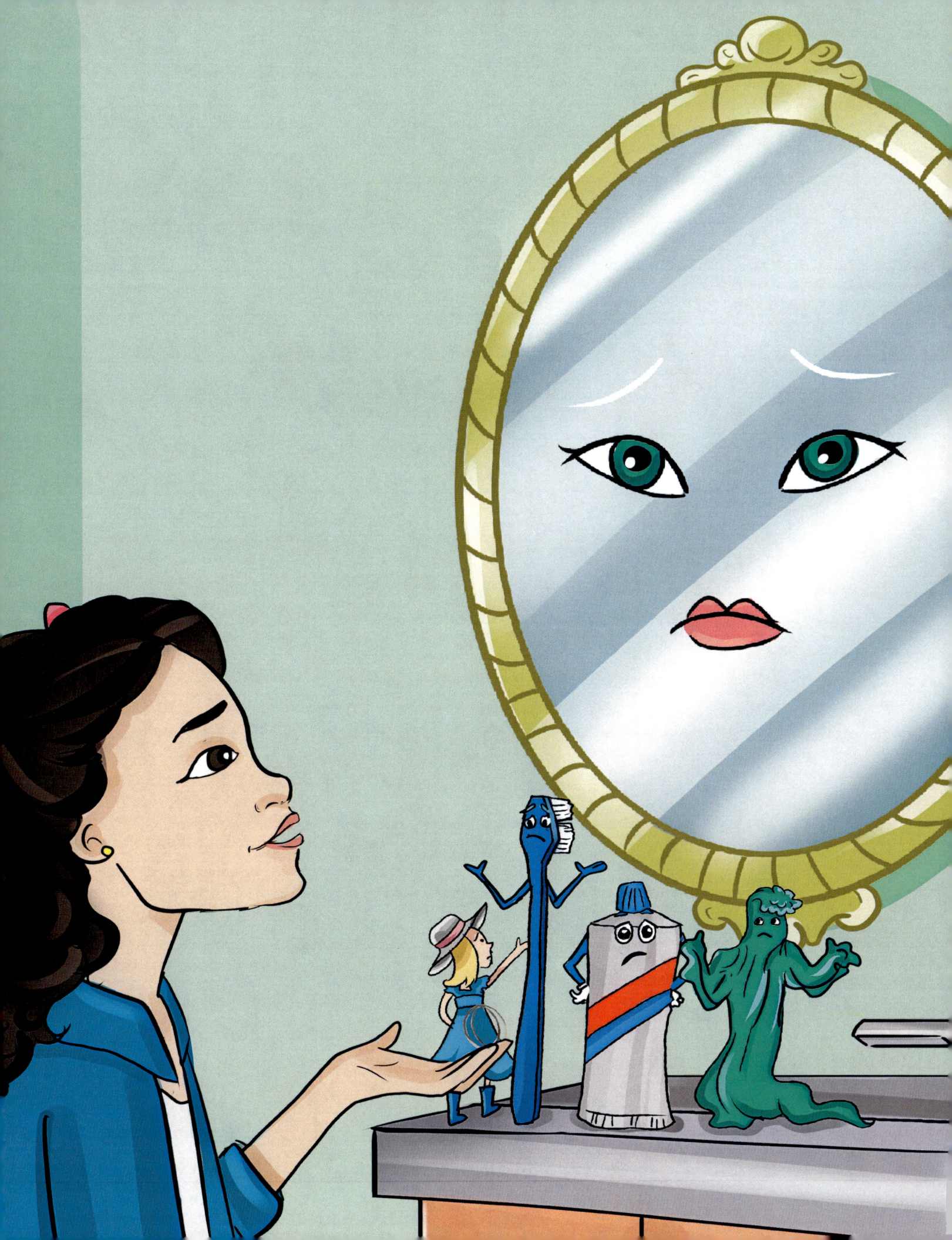

Amiya wrinkled her brow as she tried to understand.

"What is plaque and bacteria?" she asked.

"Plaque is that soft white substance that builds up on your teeth. Bacteria, the leader of the group, and his army of germs, are the worst ones of all," Brushy told Amiya.

"Why?" Amiya asked. "Bacteria and his army of germs feed on plaque," Brushy continued. "Bacteria also feed on the leftover food between your teeth, and this can cause bad breath, and even worse, cavities. So, if Anthony doesn't brush his teeth, bacteria and his army of germs will grow."

Amiya didn't like hearing this at all.

"Oh, my!" she said. "We have to get to Anthony right away. No time to waste!"

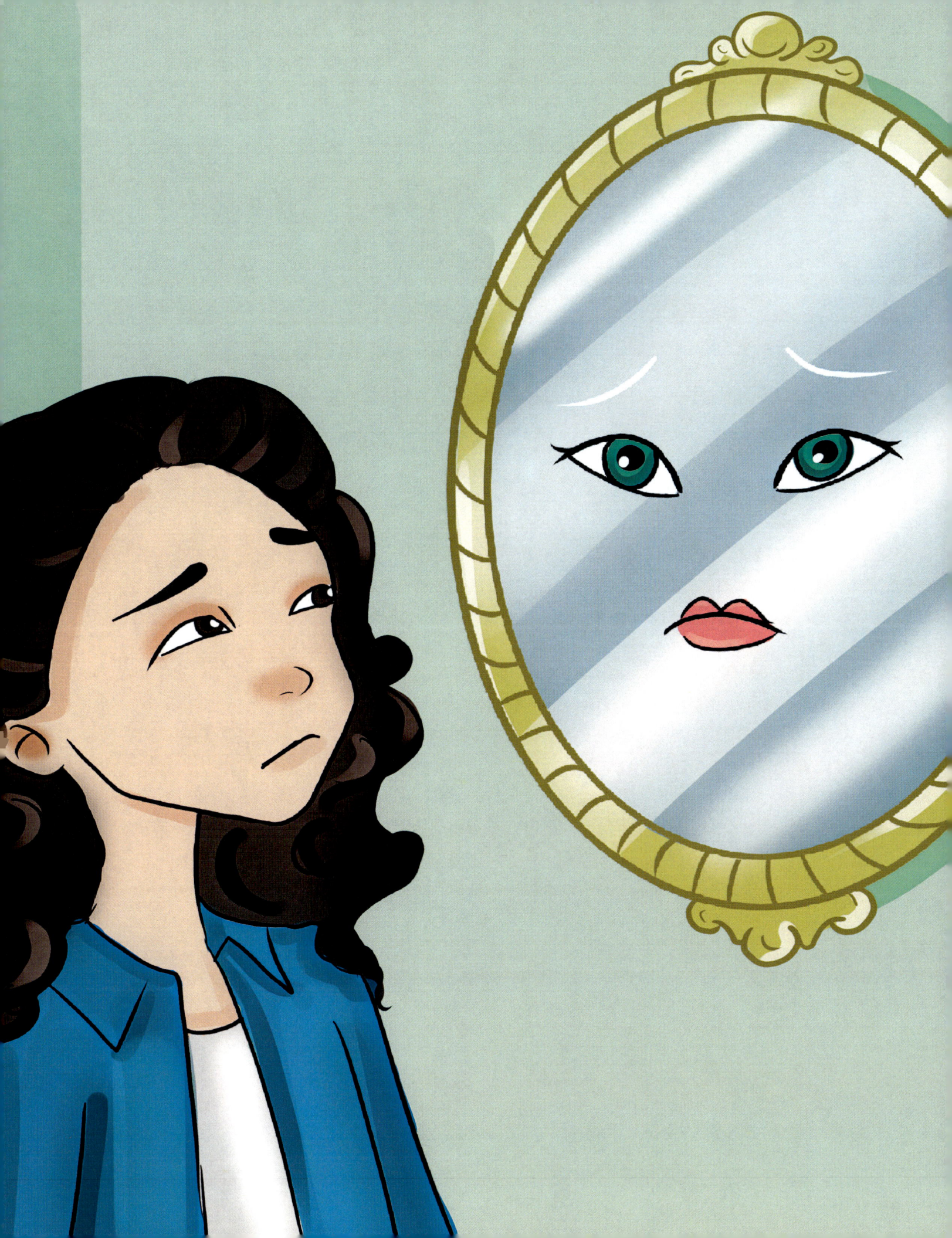

"Well, what are we waiting for?" Maggy asked.
Maggy the magical mirror started to glow brightly and then she started to sing a happy tune. Brushy began spinning his brush and Squeezy moved from side to side. Flouri the fluoride sparkled brightly and Flossy started to sparkle.
Then, Flossy let loose a huge sparkling lasso.
"I know what's next," Amiya clapped and said excitedly.
"Go Wave Go!" they all shouted.

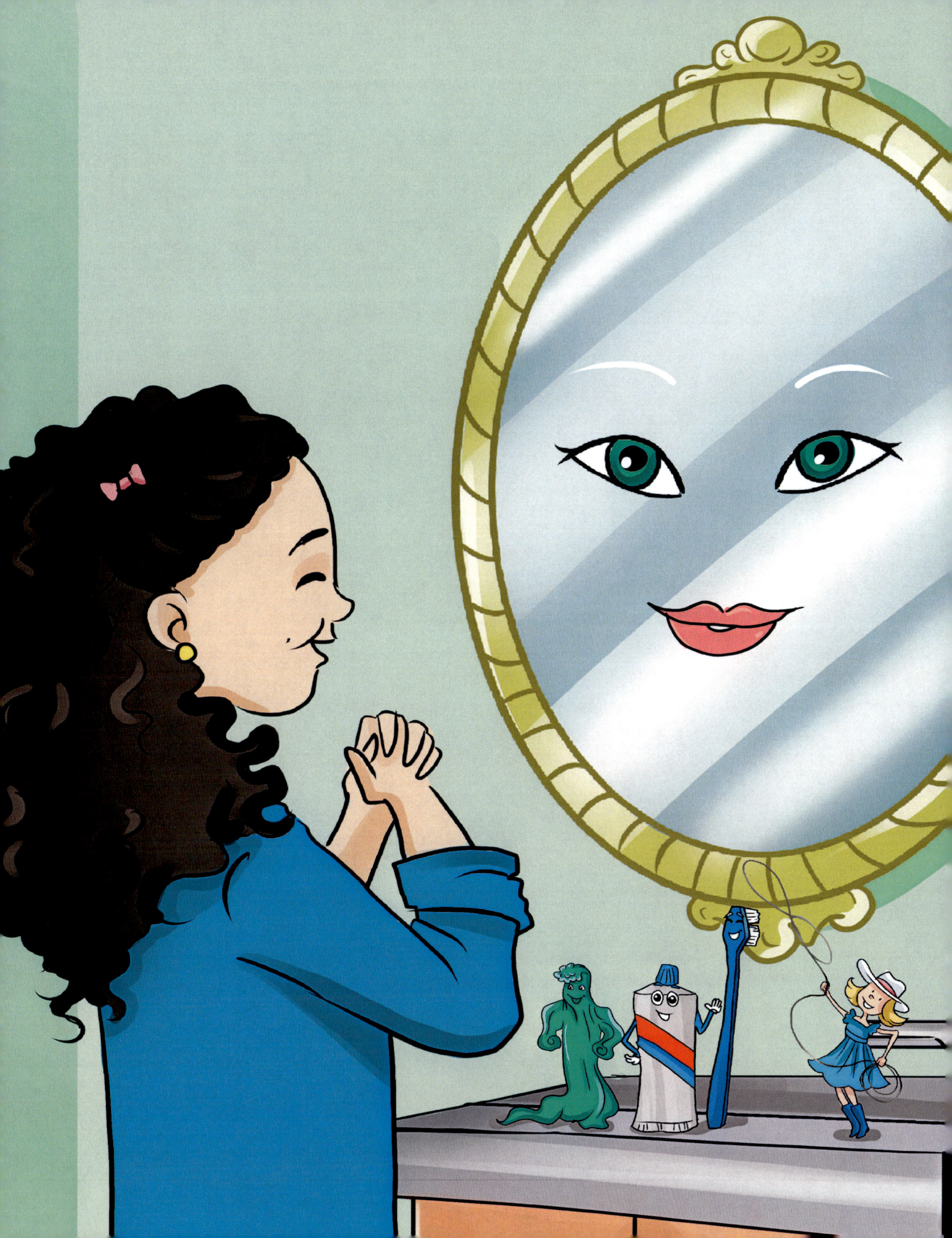

Flouri the fluoride let loose a huge wave of fluoride that picked up Amiya, Brushy and Squeezy. Flossy lassoed on as they all shouted out, "Go Mirror Go!"
They all rode the wave that took them through Maggy the magical mirror.

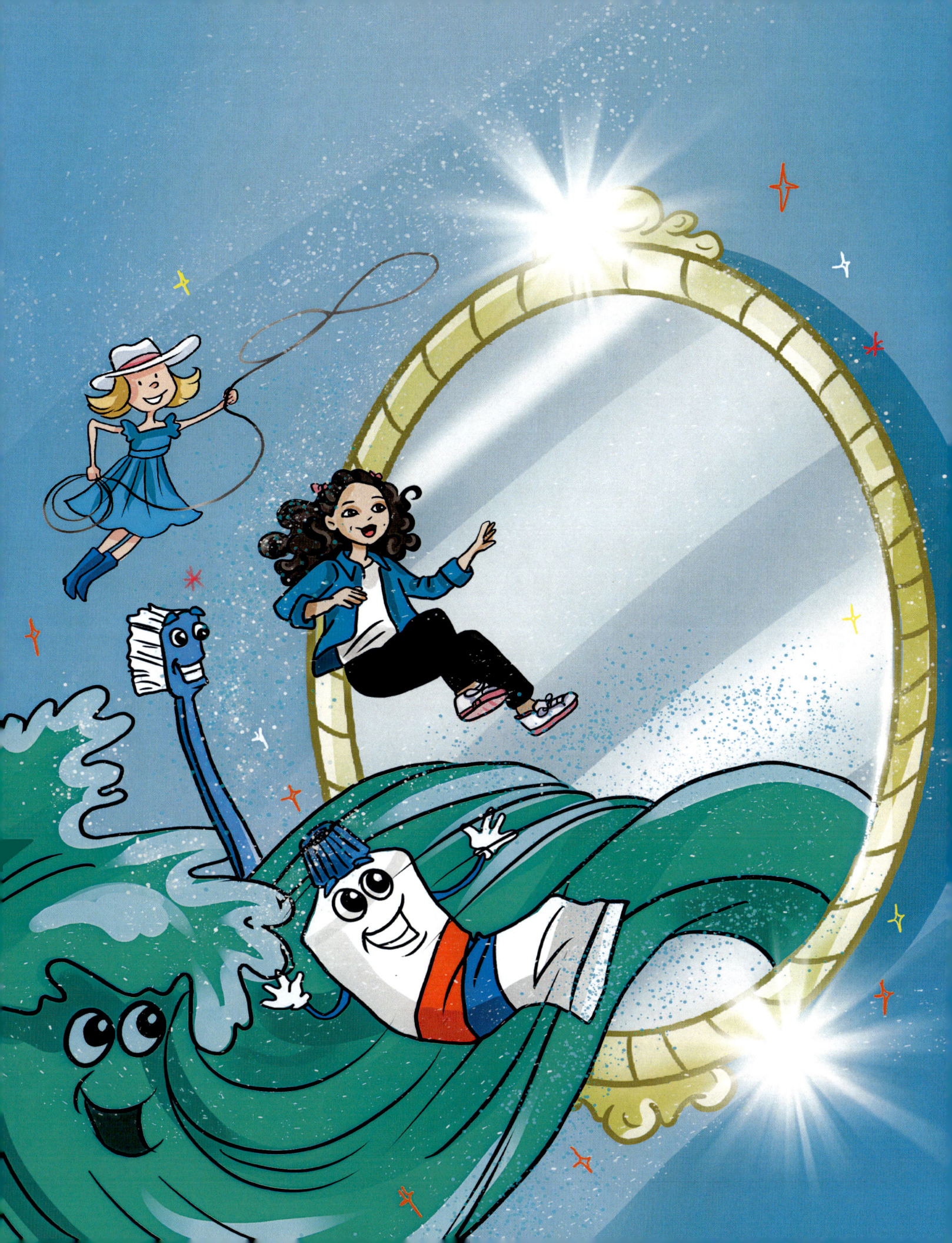

On their way to help Anthony, Flossy noticed something blocking their path.

"Phew!" they all cried.

"What is that awful smell?" Flossy asked.

"It has to be Bad Breath," Amiya said confidently. It was hard to forget what Bad Breath smelled like.

"It is Bad Breath, but he is not alone," Brushy said.

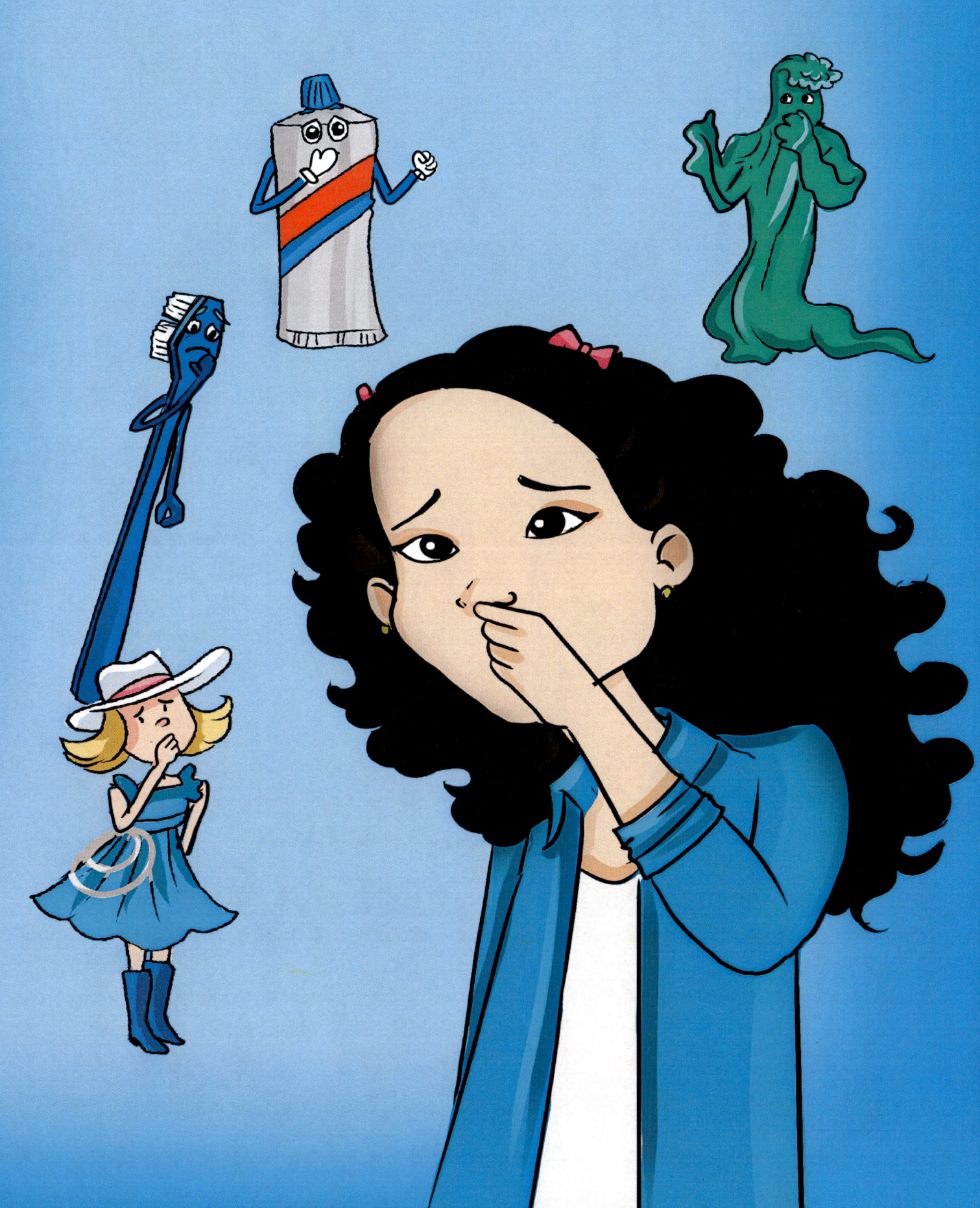

That's right," Bad Breath boasted.

"This time I brought some friends. This is Plaquey Plaque, Bacteria, and his army of germs. Ha Ha! Hee Hee!" laughed Bad Breath.

"You won't be able to win this time."

"I know all about you Bacteria," Amiya said bravely.

"We are not afraid of you or your army of germs."

Bacteria, being the leader and the smartest in the group, knew that Amiya and her friends were on their way to help Anthony to get him to brush his teeth.

He knew he had to stop them, so Bacteria ordered his army of germs and Plaquey Plaque to attack Amiya and her friends.

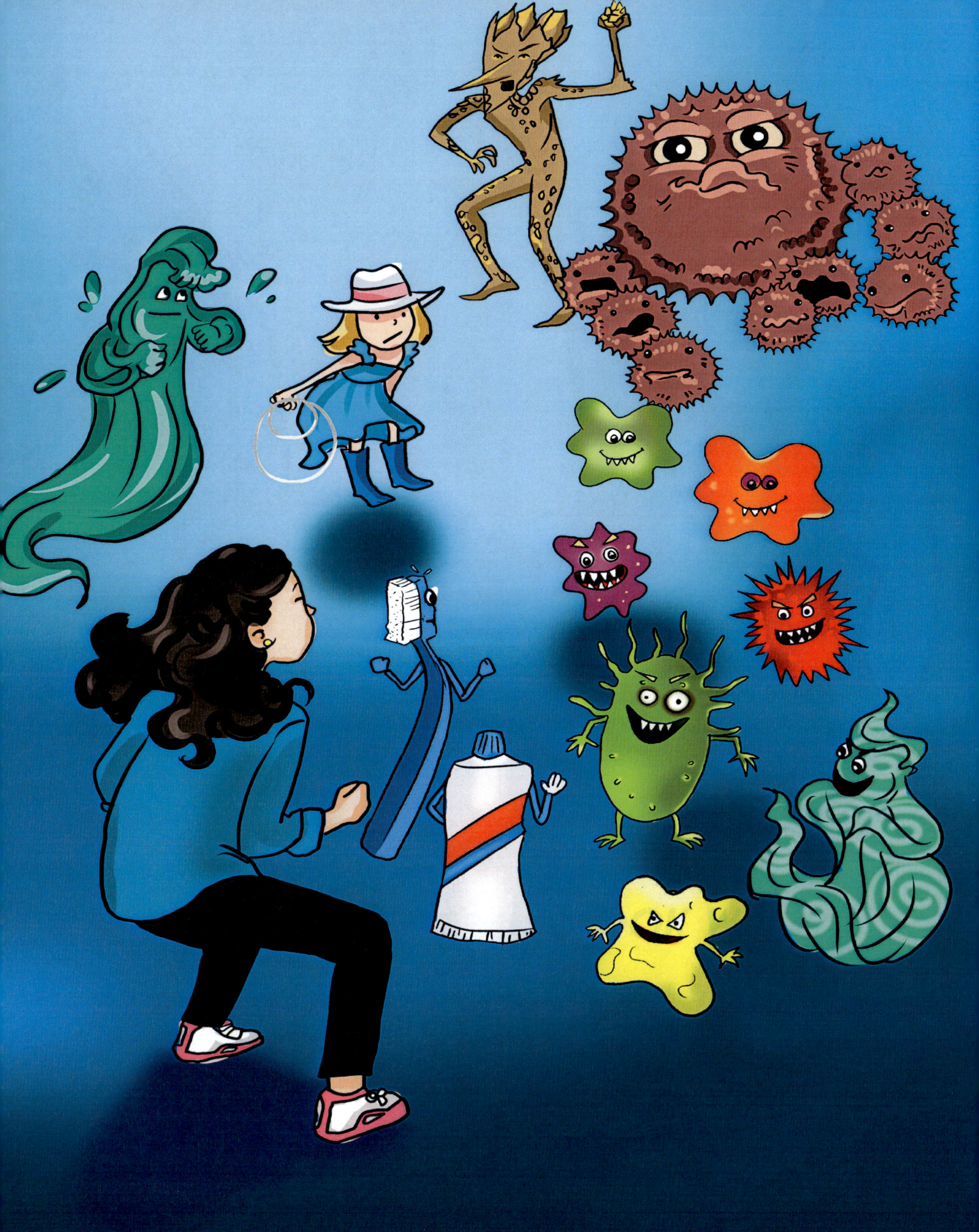

Plaquey Plaque started to throw globs of plaque at Amiya and her friends.
"AAHHHHHHHH!!!!" Amiya and her friends yelled as they ducked to escape being hit by plaque.
Then bacteria and his army of germs began to gobble down the globs of plaque and when they did, they started to grow.
The globs of plaque, germs and Bacteria headed straight for Amiya and her friends.
Bad breath thought this was very funny, so he doubled over laughing with his legs sticking in the air. "Ha Ha! Hee Hee!"
"What are we going to do?" Amiya asked.

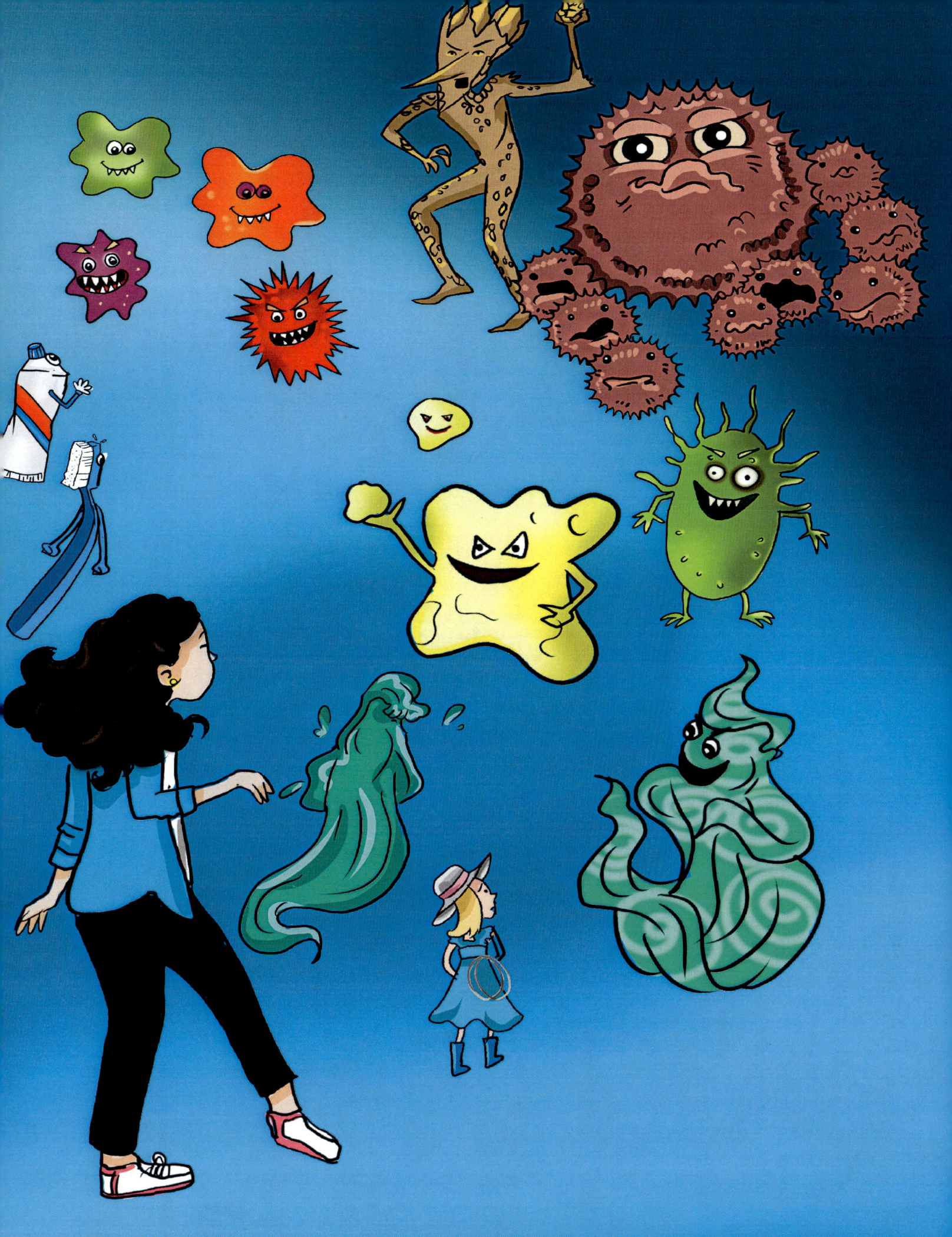

All of a sudden, Flouri the fluoride blocked the globs of plaque, bacteria, and germs with a huge wave of his fluoride. But he did not block them all. Some globs of plaque, bacteria and germs still got through. Flossy flung her lasso at the loose plaque and squeezed them until they all disappeared. Brushy spun his brush really fast, and Squeezy squeezed out his own globs of toothpaste, and together they got rid of the rest of the bacteria and germs. "Hooray! Hooray!" Amiya and her friends cheered.

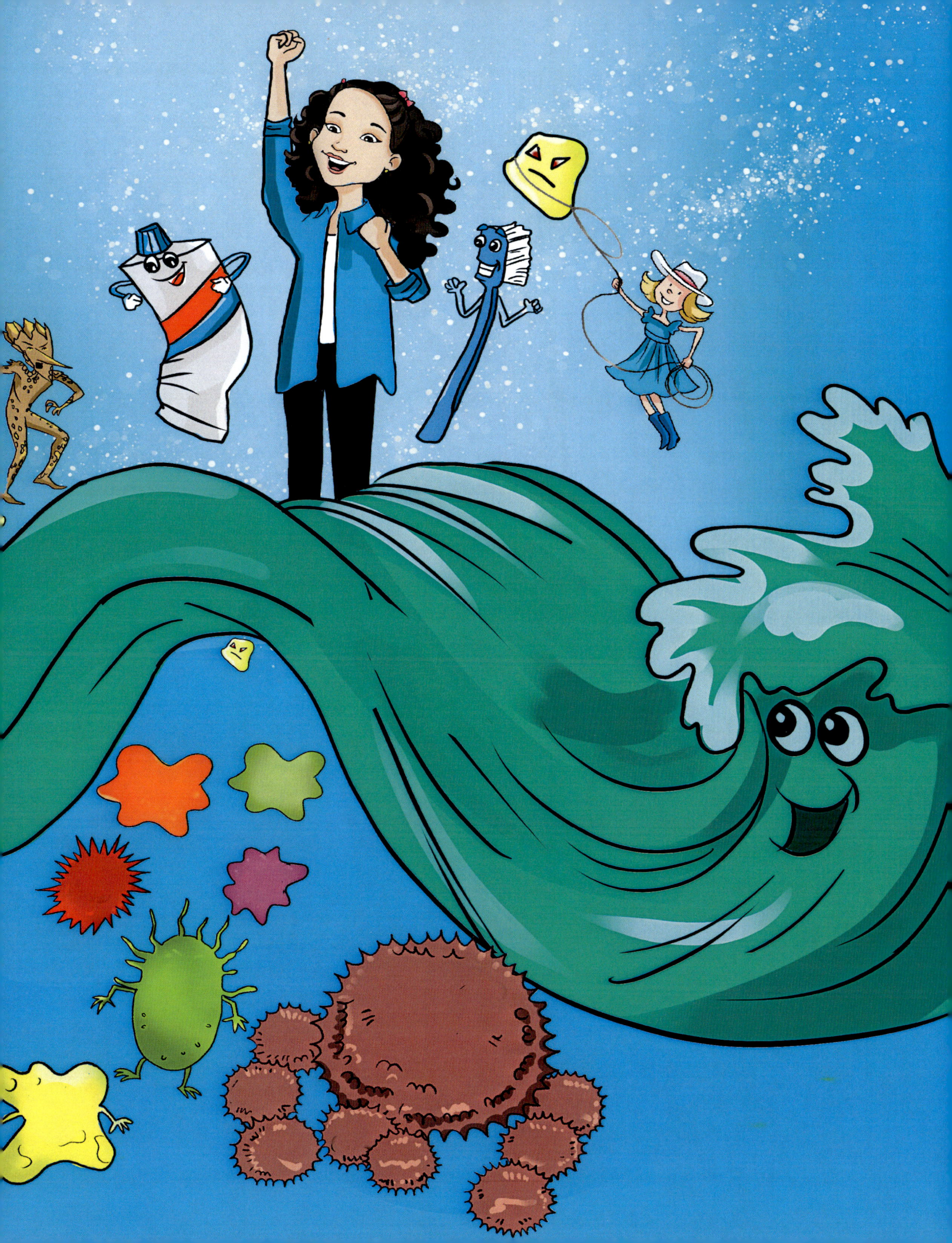

"Whew! That was close," Amiya said. "But now we have to hurry to see Anthony." "We do, but we are so tired from our battle with Plaquey Plaque, Bacteria, and his army of germs. Will you help us Amiya?" Brushy asked. "You bet I will," Amiya replied. Just then, they all shouted, "Go, Mirror, Go!" Maggy the magical mirror started to glow brightly, and they started moving again, until they were all able to see Anthony.

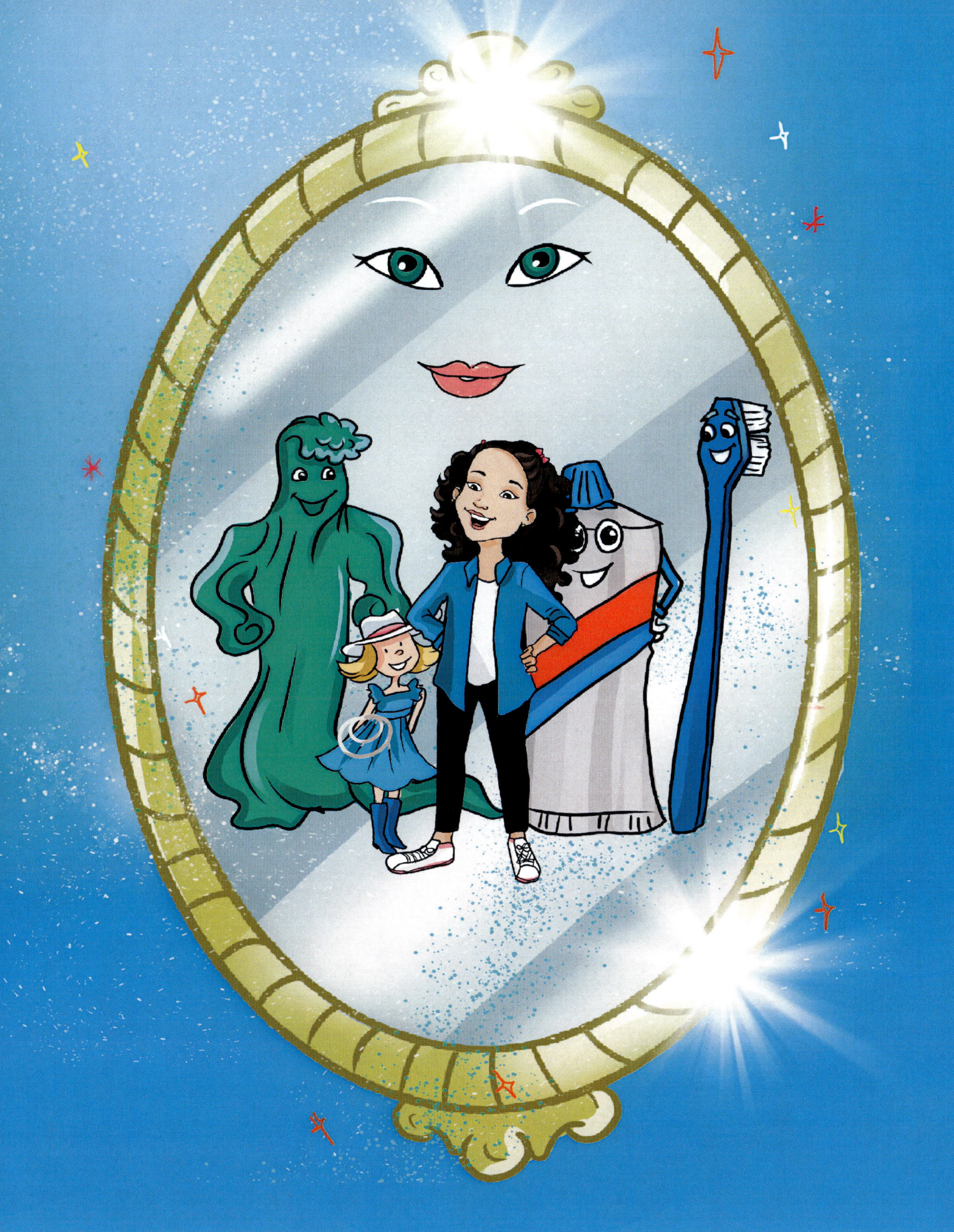

"Who are you?" Anthony asked when he saw the magical people in his mirror.

"I'm Amiya and these are my friends," Amiya told him. "This is Brushy the toothbrush, Squeezy the toothpaste, Flossy the dental floss and Flouri the fluoride."

"Hello," they all called to Anthony.

"Brushy and Squeezy work together to help keep your teeth clean," Amiya told Anthony.

"Flossy the dental floss helps to get rid of leftover food between your teeth. Flouri the fluoride helps to keep your teeth healthy and strong. And last, but not least, this is Maggy the magical mirror. She helped us to get here."

"What are you doing in my mirror?" Anthony asked.

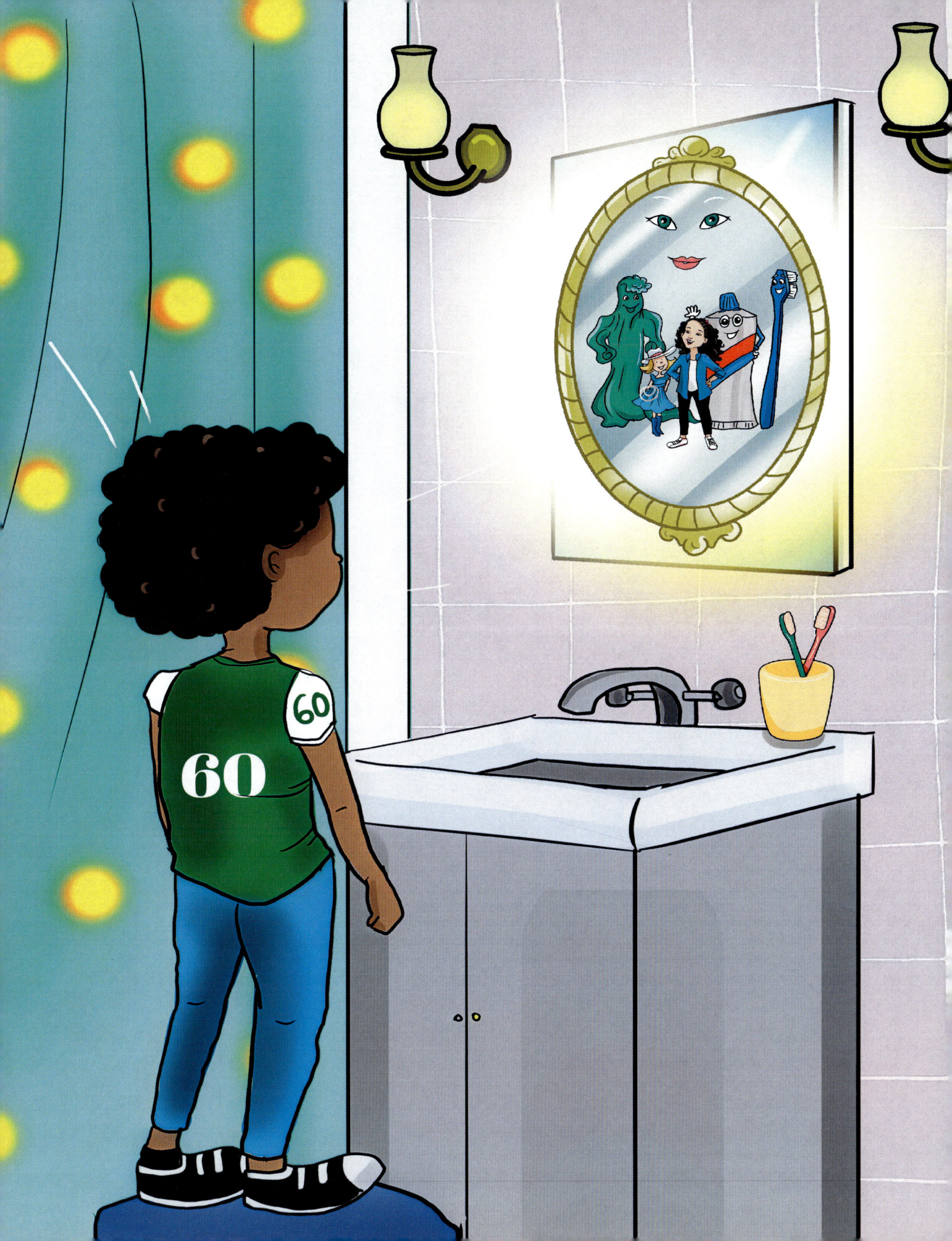

"We are all here because you did not brush your teeth today," Amiya told Anthony.

"Why do I need to brush my teeth today?" Anthony asked, with a confused look on his face. "I already brushed them last night before I went to bed!"

"No, but you have to brush them every day to fight the battle against bacteria and germs," Amiya explained.

"These bacteria and germs live in a soft white substance called plaque. Bacteria and germs feed off the plaque and the leftover food between our teeth, and that can cause bad breath, and worse, cavities. That's why you have to brush every day, once in the morning and again at night before you go to bed." "Oh," Anthony said with surprise. "I never knew that. I'm going to brush my teeth right now. I don't want that bactry to get on them."

"It's bacteria," Amiya said and giggled.

"Bacteria. Right. And I will always remember to brush my teeth once in the morning and again at night before I go to bed."

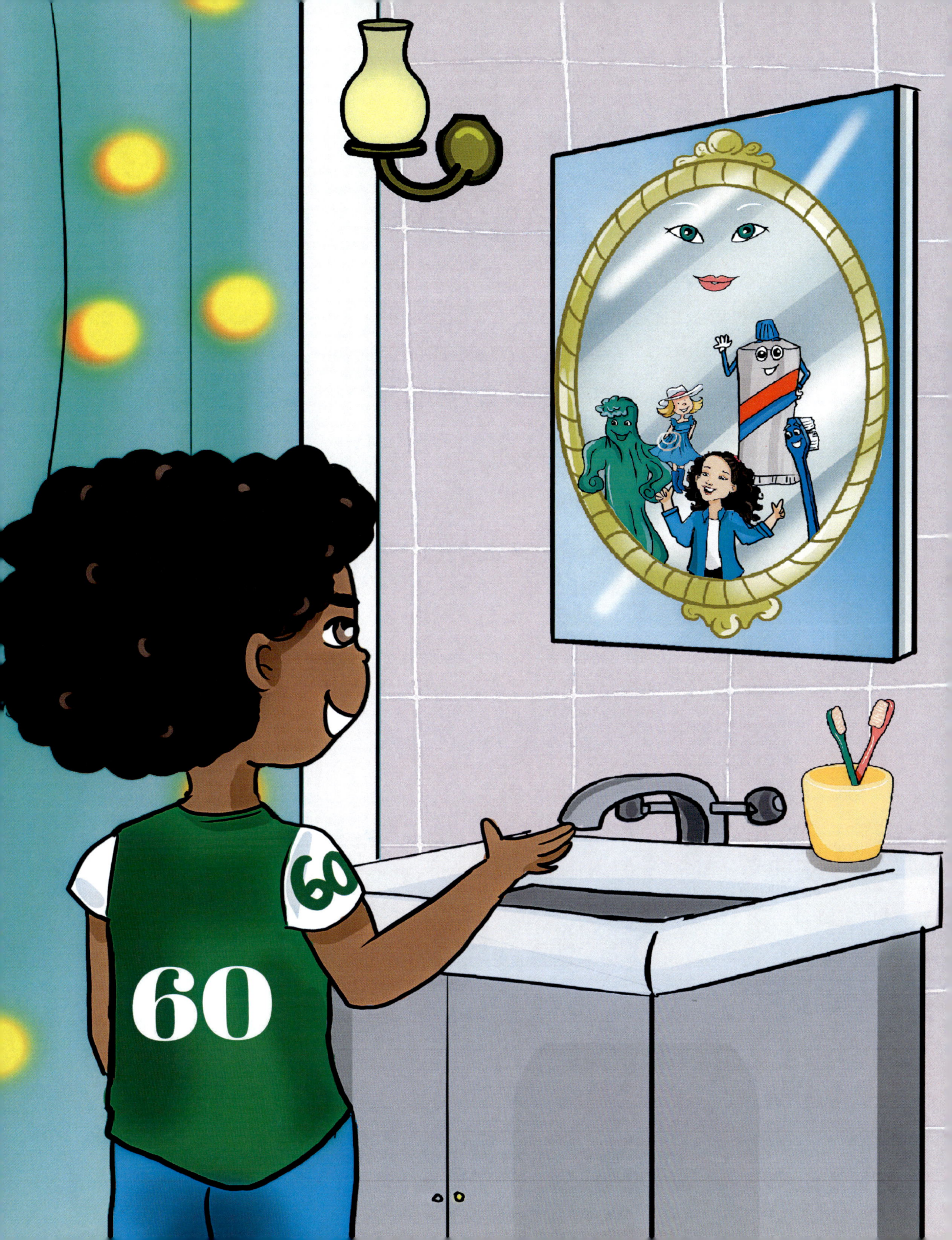

Amiya and her friends were so happy. They all started to cheer. "Hooray Anthony!"

"Before we go, I have a special gift for you," Amiya told Anthony. "This will help you to stick to your plan of brushing your teeth every day, twice a day." Amiya gave Anthony his very own Brushy the toothbrush, Squeezy the toothpaste, Flossy the dental floss and Flouri Fluoride. Anthony thanked his new friends.

"Now, we have to go. I have to get to school," Amiya said to Anthony. "Bye!" "Bye!" Anthony called back as Amiya and her friends disappeared into Maggy the mirror.

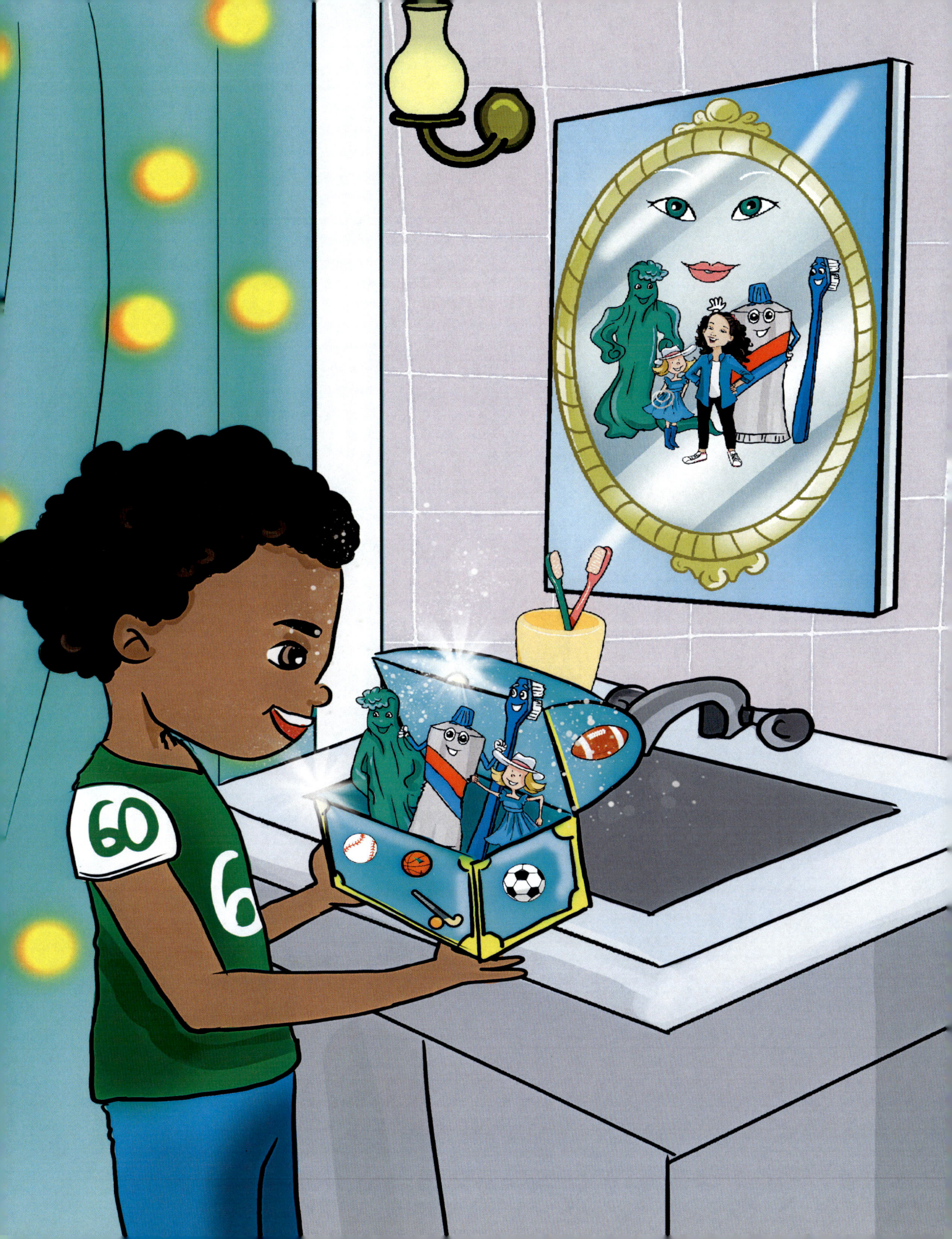

On their way back home they passed Bad Breath, Plaquey Plaque, Bacteria and his army of germs.

"You may have won this time, said Bad Breath but we'll be back. You hear me? We'll be back!" he cried and shook his fist in the air.

"We will be ready for you"! Amiya shouted back.

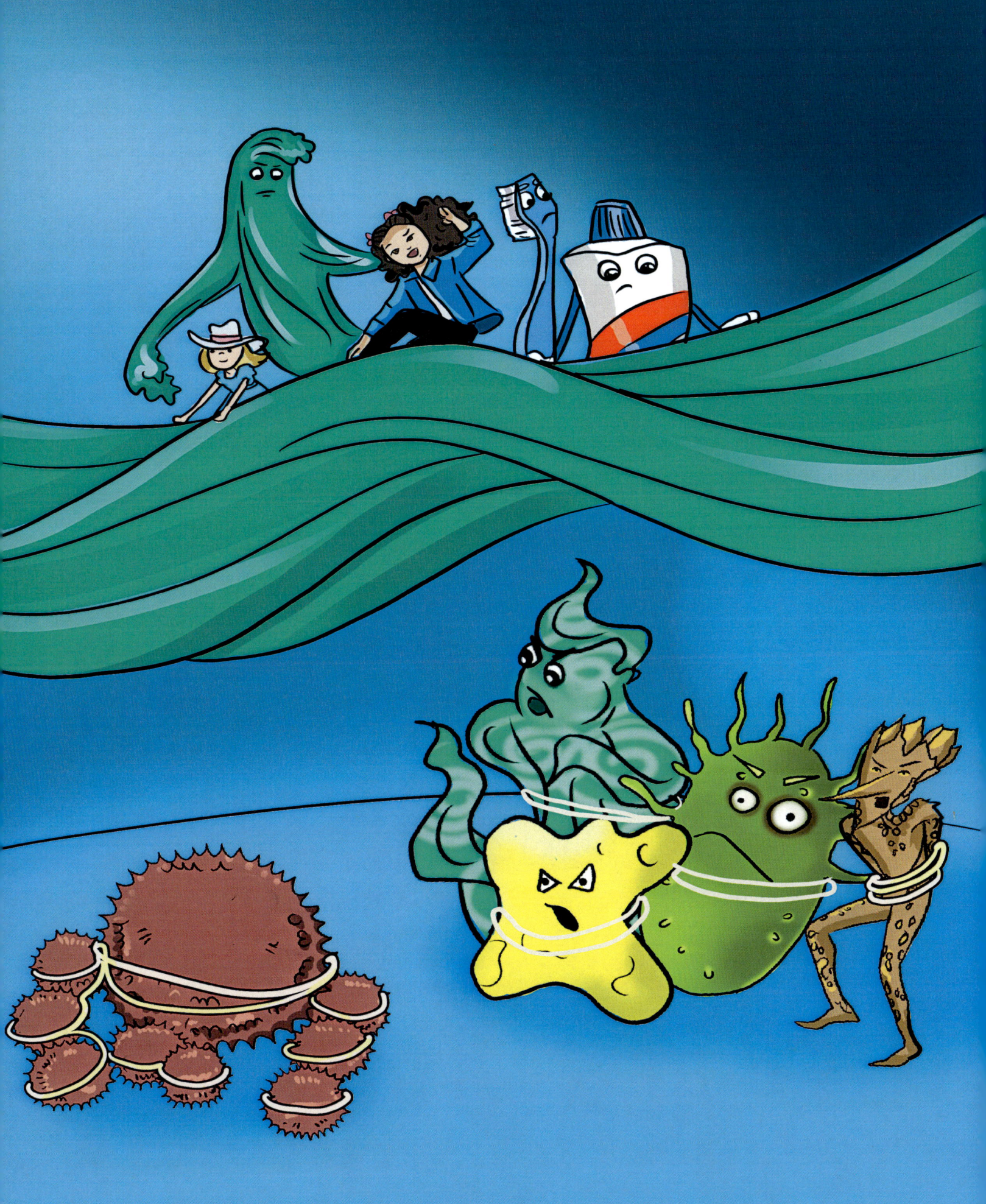

Just then there was a flash, and Amiya found herself back home and in her bathroom.

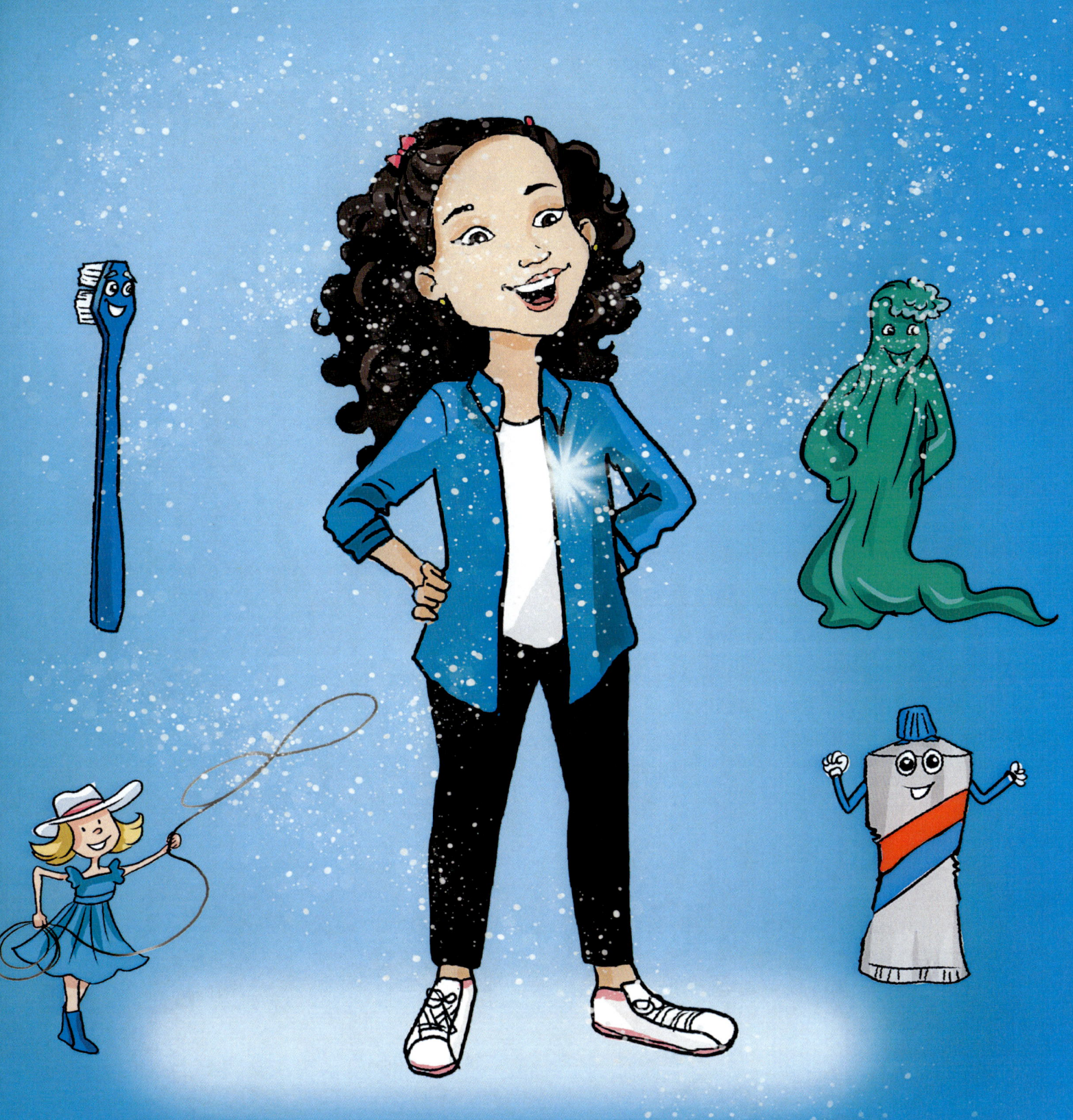

You did a really good job today," Brushy told Amiya as she stood once more in her bathroom. "I couldn't have done it without you," she told them. "See you soon," Brushy said as they all jumped back into the magical box. Amiya smiled and waved goodbye to all of her friends before putting her magical box away. She was already looking forward to seeing them again later that night when it will be time to brush again!

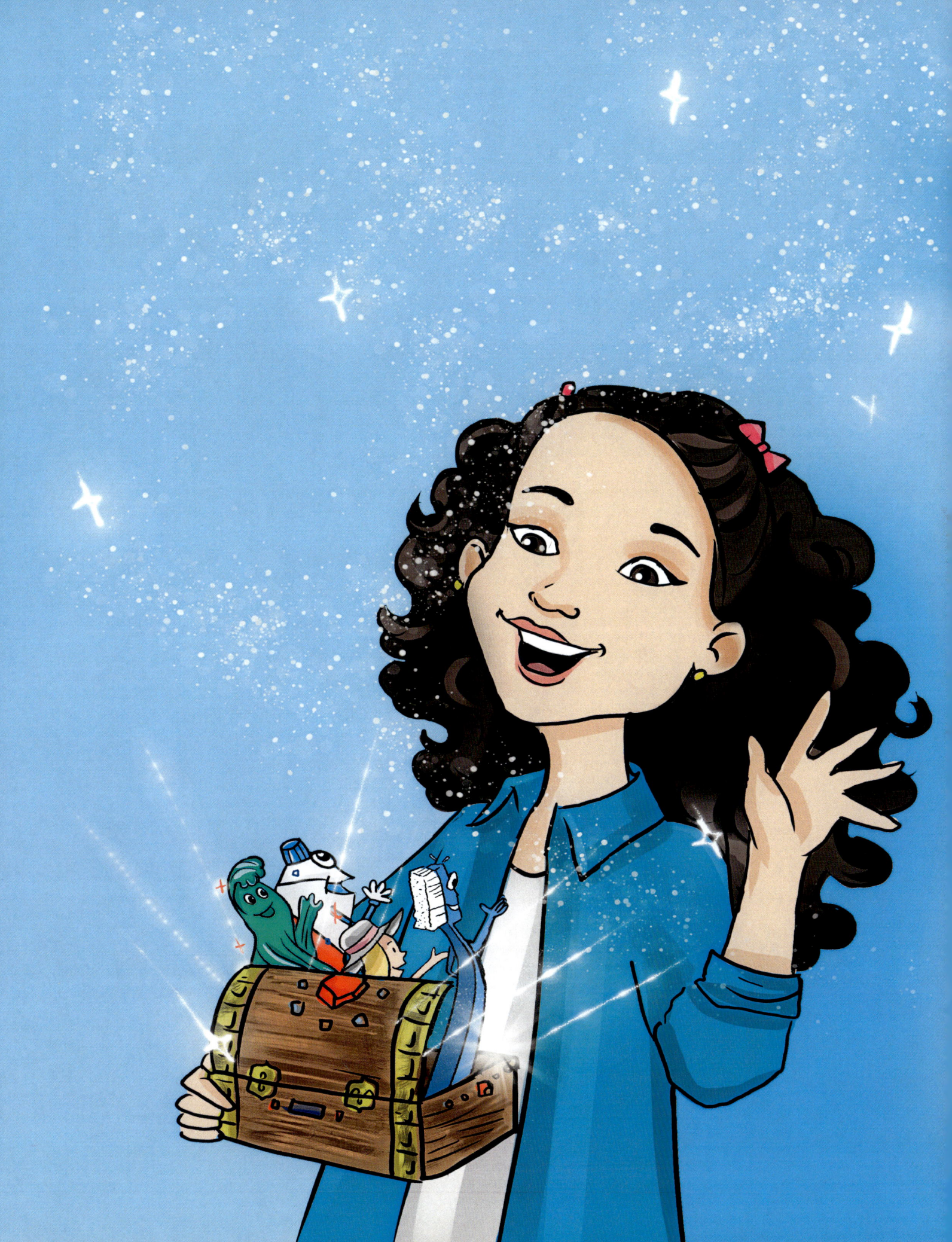

Made in United States
North Haven, CT
11 November 2022

26611560R00024